Health Advice
For My Grandchildren

Leland M. Walker

LELAND M. WALKER

DEDICATION

I dedicate this book to Tuxedo the cat. He never eats sugar.

LELAND M. WALKER

Contents

LELAND M. WALKER

Acknowledgements

Thanks to my wife, Pat, for her help with proofreading and editing.

Thanks to Jennie Houser, a long time friend who went to college with Pat. We have her wedding gift hanging over our bed. Jennie proofread several times finding many errors. She also made many suggestions for improving the flow and readability. All of her suggestions (five and one-half pages, 8.5 X 11, single spaced) have been incorporated.

Thanks to Norma Bruce for offering to help with the proofreading. Norma was our neighbor in Jonesboro for years and remains one of our best friends. Norma's many suggestions and corrections are incorporated.

Thanks to my daughter, Tracey, for her encouragement and proofreading. Tracey is an enthusiastic supporter of giving up sugar.

Thanks to Dr. Ferrol Sams III, Md, for keeping me alive and happy. I have excellent healthcare.

1. Purpose

"It is our choices... that show what we truly are, far more than our abilities."

- J. K. Rowling, English author (1965-present)

My Advice

Don't eat sugar.

Control your cholesterol.

Don't diet.

Exercise regularly.

Drive safely.

Know your family health history.

Get professional healthcare.

This book is about enjoying life. The implication is that by the decisions you make and by the way you live, you can do something about (1) how you feel, (2) which diseases you get, and (3) how long you live. I choose to believe in Free Will. The Destiny philosophy doesn't give you much motivation to do anything.

This book is about adopting a lifestyle that balances work and play. Adopt a lifestyle that includes daily sacrifices for future rewards. Strive for continuous improvement. Be a little better tomorrow than you are today. Have a five year plan. Measure your progress. The things you measure are the things you improve. It takes work and luck, but I have found that the harder I work the luckier I get. Be like Benjamin Franklin and W. Edwards Deming.

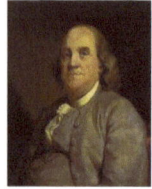

Ben Franklin

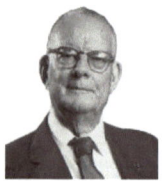

W. Edwards Deming

2. Sugar

My Advice

Give up sugar.

Do not eat food that has any kind of sugar listed as an added ingredient (lactose, dextrose, maltose, corn syrup, etc.)

Do not eat any food that has more than 3 grams of natural sugar per serving (this includes milk and fruit juice.)

Sugar is today what cigarettes were when I was young. Sugar is harmful to our health and it has a powerful industry telling us it is not. The consumption of sugar in our country is very slowly on the decline and has been for about 15 years. We are making progress. But it tastes so good and the harmful effects are not immediately apparent so denial is very easy.

I have type II diabetes.

In 2005 I was diagnosed as a type II diabetic. Following my routine physical, my doctor informed me I had high blood sugar due to insulin resistance. This was based on my A1C (hemoglobin A1c) results. A1C is a blood test that gives an indication of your average blood sugar level for the previous three months by assessing glycated hemoglobin.

"A normal A1C level is 5.6 percent or below, according to the National Institute of Diabetes and Digestive and Kidney Diseases. A level of 5.7 to 6.4 percent indicates prediabetes, and people with diabetes have an A1C level at 6.5 percent or above."[1]

My A1C was above 7.0. My doctor prescribed pioglitazone (Actos®) twice daily "to help with the insulin uptake." I was also given a prescription for a blood sugar monitoring device. I began pricking my finger every morning before I ate to measure my fasting blood sugar.

I was scheduled for follow-up visits every 6 months. I followed my doctor's instructions for about a year.

I was already on a regular exercise schedule. I did not vary from my exercise routine. I went to the gym three to five times per week and played golf once or twice a week, walking and carrying my clubs.

Checking my blood sugar every morning reinforced my awareness of my sugar intake. My goal was blood sugar readings of 104 mg/dl (milligrams per deciliter) or less. My blood sugar was usually a little over that, but rarely above 130. After some months of not getting my blood sugar down to my goal, I decided to take sugar out of my diet.

I read the labels of everything I ate. In the ingredients list, if sugar was one the ingredients, I did not eat it. In the "Nutrition Facts" label, if natural sugar was greater than 3 grams per serving, I did not eat it. Milk and juice were out.

---

[1] *Erica Manfred, www.healthline.com/health/type-2-diabetes/ac1-test#how-it-works3, 4-22-2018.*

I think it is important to point out that giving up sugar was not all that hard to do. It was not nearly as hard as giving up cigarettes. I found that if I start the day without sugar, I don't crave sweets. It is only after I have eaten something with sugar in it that in an hour or so I get a strong craving for sweets. That craving is then never satisfied, no matter how much I eat. The trick is to never start. I will have more on hypoglycemia later.

> "For someone without diabetes, a fasting blood sugar on awakening should be under 100 mg/dl. Before-meal normal sugars are 70–99 mg/dl. "Postprandial" sugars taken two hours after meals should be less than 140 mg/dl."[2]

Within two months after I gave up sugar, my morning fasting blood sugar checks came under my goal of 104 mg/dl.

After a few months of less than 104 mg/dl fasting blood sugar, I reduced my my Actos® pills to one per day. My morning blood sugar results did not change.

On my next follow-up with my doctor, my A1C results were normal. I told my doctor that I was taking only one pill per day and he said: "OK, keep it up. You seem to be doing fine." So I quit taking the other pill. My morning blood sugar checks did not change. The readings were still always under 104.

---

[2] David Spero, BSN, RN, January 13, 2016, www.diabetesselfmanagement.com/blog/what-is-a-normal-blood-sugar-level, 3-21-2018.

Six months later my A1C results were still normal. I told my doctor about not taking the medication. His response was: "So you are controlling your diabetes with diet and exercise. Good."

Now I check my blood sugar about once every week or two in the morning before I eat. It is always under 100. It is usually between 80 and 90.

When I gave up sugar, I lost a pound per month for 30 months. I did not diet. I did not increase my exercise. I ate anything I wanted (I didn't want sugar). My weight went from 220 lb. to 190 lb. I continued to drink beer and eat bread, my two favorite foods.

Based on my experience I believe insulin resistance is reversible by giving up sugar. LP-IR is an indicator of insulin resistance that is obtained in NMR analysis of lipoproteins in the blood. My LP-IR score in October 2015 was 51. In February 2018 it was 40. The reference (goal) is <=45.

Insulin resistance marker percentile distribution of the general population:

Low	25th	50th	75th	High
<27	27	45	63	>63

<—sensitive   resistant—>

.

Sugar is poison.

The definition of "poison":

"1   a : a substance that through its chemical action usually kills, injures, or impairs an organism

b (1) : something destructive or harmful   (2) : an object of aversion or abhorrence"[3]

The negative effects of sugar on the human body are very gradual, so gradual that the effects are not associated with cause. Resistance of body tissue to insulin uptake doesn't exhibit itself until after 20 or 30 years of abuse. Damage to capillaries and blood flow by excess sugar in the blood also takes years to manifest itself, probably exacerbated by the onset of insulin resistance.

There are two categories of insulin injections. One is a slow-release and the other is quicker-acting. The slow-release is used with a strategy of controlling blood sugar by carefully controlling the calorie intake by eating small portions of carefully chosen foods and eating on a very strict schedule.

The quicker-acting type is used in a strategy of controlling blood sugar where you give yourself an injection with meals. In practice, this turns out to be eating what you want when you want and then neutralizing the sugar with an injection. People using this strategy will eat cake or pie or ice cream and give themselves an injection. They take a good helping of poison and then take the antidote.

---

[3] Merriam-Webster.com, 3-21-2018.

My brother, Marvin, wasn't fat when he was a kid. He got fat in his late teens. He became diabetic when he was a young man. He ate anything he wanted and as much as he wanted. When he got diabetes he continued to eat candy bars and anything else he wanted. He took insulin. To me it seemed like he ate the poison and then injected the antidote. Well that didn't work out so well. His diabetes caused his kidneys to fail. He lived a long time considering he was on insulin and dialysis for a significant part of his life. He died in his early sixties. I am a little mad at him for not giving up the candy bars.

Humans evolved without concentrated sugar.

For the general population, refined sugar has been around for only a few hundred years. The wealthy and royal have had access to sugar a few centuries longer. But on the scale of our evolution, sugar has just arrived. As a result, the human body is unable to handle even moderate amounts of pure sugar.

Hypoglycemia signals a problem with insulin.

When you eat complex carbs the digestion process is slow. It takes a long time for the gut to break down the carbs and free up the sugars. The blood sugar levels come up very slowly, and the body slowly supplies just the right amount of insulin to handle it. We evolved on just such a diet, and the body knows what to do.

When you eat refined sugar or natural sugars in high concentrations, the body is not capable of handling it.

Your blood sugar level jumps quickly to unhealthy levels. My cousin Wayne said his blood sugar has been as high as 300 mg/dl. These are the levels where organs are damaged.

Then, the body dumps insulin...too much. The insulin binds with the sugar so the body can absorb it. In an hour or two the sugar is all bound to insulin and you will have free insulin left over. Excess insulin causes tissues to become insulin resistant. Also, these are the conditions where low blood sugar makes you feel weak and shaky. You then get the uncontrollable urge to eat some sugar.

You are on the hypoglycemic roller coaster, and you will stay on it until you go to bed and sleep it off. Tomorrow is another day. You can try again, without sugar.

I will not spend a lot more time re-writing all the reasons not to eat sugar. The work has already been done. If you want to read about it I recommend:

"The Case Against Sugar" by Gary Taubes. If you want more convincing, Gary Taubes' book has a very extensive bibliography.

"Sweet Poison: Why Sugar Makes Us Fat," by David Gillespie. David Gillespie has written several books on the subject of sugar.

Sugar is the new tobacco. The data is in. But for the general public, reducing sugar intake is going to be a lot more difficult than giving up cigarettes. It is going to take the passing of several generations to convince the general public. Even then, there will always be a large percentage of the population that will continue to eat it. Just consider how many people still smoke cigarettes.

Sugar is such an important part of our lives. It is added to a very large part of our processed food. For example, only shredded wheat, and one of the Fiber One® cereals do not have sugar as an ingredient. The original Cheerios®

Is not too bad with 1 gram per ounce. All the rest are pretty much just candy. The entire cereal aisle is candy. It tastes so good, and there are no immediate ill effects.

It has not been proven that sugar causes diabetes.

In this book I write about type II, late onset diabetes. Type I diabetes is a completely different matter, and I have no advice on the subject.

When I was growing up we called it "sugar diabetes." We didn't know there was a type I and type II. My mother would say: "You're gonna get sugar diabetes if you don't quit eating all that candy." I knew better. I knew that diabetes is when your pancreas doesn't make enough insulin. Now I have to say I think she was right. I *do believe* that type II diabetes is caused by purified and concentrated sugar.

In history, whenever a society began to consume refined sugar there followed an epidemic of type II diabetes. Before sugar became a significant part of our diet type II diabetes was nonexistent. See "The Case Against Sugar" by Gary Taubes for a thorough discussion of the correlation.

The AMA (American Medical Association) currently holds the position that the increase in the occurrence of diabetes is the result of the increase in obesity, and that the increase in obesity is the result of the increase of fats and carbohydrates in our diets. They place a lot of significance on the role increased sugar plays in the increase in obesity, but they stop short of saying sugar causes diabetes.

There doesn't seem to be any study that shows a direct cause/effect relation between sugar and diabetes. Oh, there are plenty of studies that show the *correlation* between sugar consumption and diabetes, but correlation is not cause/effect.

The correlation of increase sugar consumption with exponential increase of diabetes is not enough for the AMA to take on the food industry. Think tobacco. I remember the years of struggle to get a general acceptance that cigarettes cause lung cancer. It is going to be a long time before the general population accepts that sugar causes diabetes. The food industry is so strong and sugar tastes so good. I really doubt it will happen in my lifetime.

We really need controlled studies to show the physiological effects of sugar on non-diabetics, and the effect of sugar on a fetus. I admit my search of the literature has been very limited to this point, but I have not found any studies of this nature.

I hypothesize that refined sugar in the diet causes diabetes. I am suggesting that in the time it takes for the body to neutralize and use raw sugar, probably a couple of hours, two things happen:

1. **Insulin resistance develops.** Hypoglycemia (the result of overcompensation of the body to high blood sugar) occurs when the body produces insulin to control the excess sugar in the blood. The body can't handle a sudden increase in blood sugar. It will try to neutralize the sugar but it will overcompensate. It takes about an hour or two to pump out enough insulin to handle the sugar in a candy bar or a soda. By then there is an excess of insulin in the blood. The body then craves sugar to restore blood sugar to normal levels. The cycle repeats. During these periods of excess insulin, the body compensates by the muscles beginning to acquire a resistance to insulin. Based on my own experience, I believe this acquired insulin resistance is reversible to some degree with a sugar-free diet.

2. **Capillaries are damaged.** Damage occurs to circulation in the eyes, internal organs, and extremities. Diabetics are at risk for circulatory problems. This is the result of high blood sugar. During the hour or so it takes for the body to produce the insulin to metabolize refined sugar, why would the body not undergo the same conditions experienced by a diabetic when their blood sugar is not controlled? I suggest (and I believe) repeated short durations of high blood sugar, several times per day, every day, could have a cumulative damaging effect on organs, perhaps even the organs that produce insulin.

As with cigarettes, efforts to reduce sugar consumption are going to meet resistance from the industry that produces the foods that contain sugar.

For example, the International Life Sciences Institute. (Its members include Coca-Cola, Hershey, Red-Bull, Oreo cookie maker Mondelez, and Mars Inc) funded a paper

> "...that says global recommendations on limiting sugar are based on weak evidence." It is encouraging that Mars Inc., a member of the funding group, joined in the criticism of this paper. Mars said: "...the paper undermines the work of public health officials and makes all industry-funded research look bad." The Mars spokesperson went on to say: "...even Mars realizes people consume too much sugar, and wants to help them understand how to cut back."[4]

There is more evidence of progress in the reduction of sugar consumption in the US. The annual consumption of sugar in the US peaked in 1999 at 155 lb. per person. In 2014 sugar consumption was 114 lb. per person.[5]

The reduction is encouraging, but dang! That is a lot of sugar.

---

[4] The Miami Herald, International Edition, December 23, 2016, pages 2a and 2b

[5] Gary Taubes, *The Case Against Sugar*

Here are some symptoms of diabetes.

This list of symptoms came from the source noted. The descriptions are my re-writes. Some of the information came from other places.[6]

1. Numbness in the extremities is often the first sign of diabetes in adults. This is the result of reduced blood flow in the small blood vessels and the resulting damage to nerve cells. The numbness would feel like a pricky or tingly pain that progresses slowly, perhaps over several years.

2. Frequent urination is also an early sign of type II diabetes, and is often the trigger for a diagnosis. The kidneys are flushing the excess sugar from the blood. This can easily result in dehydration. Dehydration can lead to other illnesses, the most serious being kidney failure. If you're a diabetic and you eat sugar, you better drink a lot of water...like 3 liters or more per day.

3. Weight loss, unexplained by changes in diet or exercise, can be the result of your body not processing glucose properly. You might not have enough insulin (type I diabetes). But it is more likely your muscle tissue has acquired a resistance to insulin (type II diabetes) after years of fluctuation between high blood sugar and low blood sugar (excess insulin). Remember the hypoglycemia roller coaster. With all your glucose going out through your kidneys your body has to start burning fat and muscle to get energy and you lose weight.

4. Increase in appetite might follow or accompany the weight loss, which seems logical. You are not getting enough nourishment to maintain your weight.

---

[6] Catherine Roberts, 7-12-2013, www.activebeat.co/your-health/10-common-symptoms-of-diabetes, 3-21-2018.

5. Blurry vision can result from damage to the retina by the poor circulation.

6. Itchy, dry skin results from poor circulation to the sweat glands.

7. Unexplained fatigue results from poor circulation, poor nutrition, and muscle deterioration.

8. Unquenchable thirst results from the frequent urination and dehydration.

9. Slow healing cuts or bruises results from the poor blood flow to wounds and from a general deterioration of the immune system.

10. Irritated gums is a two way street...the poor circulation can lead to periodontal disease which can add to the total inflammation in the body, exacerbating the diabetes symptoms.

The following chart is a plot of my blood sugar over the course of one day. You will see the normal fluctuation of blood sugar before and after meals. This is how it is supposed to look when the body is maintaining proper control of blood sugar.

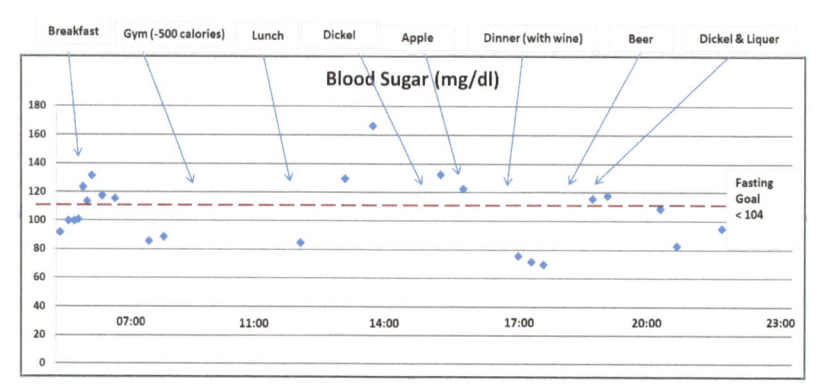

3. Cholesterol

My Advice

Don't be fat.

Keep your cholesterol within recommended guidelines.

Follow up high cholesterol with a lipid profile.

Take statins because diet won't do it.

The main points I want to promote in this chapter are:

- High LDL cholesterol causes artery blockage.
- Artery blockage causes heart disease and strokes.
- High cholesterol is more a result of who you are than what you eat.
- You can prevent the artery blockage that is caused by high LDL cholesterol.

What is cholesterol?

Cholesterol: The most common type of steroid in the body. Cholesterol has a reputation for being associated with an increased risk for heart and blood vessel disease. However, cholesterol is essential to the formation of bile acids, vitamin D, progesterone, estrogens (estradiol, estrone, estriol), androgens (androsterone, testosterone), mineralocorticoid hormones (aldosterone, corticosterone), and glucocorticoid hormones (cortisol). Cholesterol is also necessary to the normal permeability and function of the membranes that surround cells. A diet high in saturated fats tends to increase blood cholesterol levels, whereas a diet high in unsaturated fats tends to lower blood cholesterol levels. Although some cholesterol is obtained from the diet, most cholesterol is made in the liver and other tissues. The treatment of elevated cholesterol involves not only diet but also weight loss, regular exercise, and medications. After the age of 20, cholesterol testing is recommended every 5 years.[7]

I have heart problems.

After I retired from DuPont I went back to school at Virginia Tech to study physics and math. I was in my 4th semester, 15 minutes into Partial Differential Equations class, when I experienced my first angina. It was not painful. It was just a strange feeling in my chest that I had never felt before. The best description I can come up with is a "pressure" or "tightness" just left of the sternum. That was in the spring of 1997. I was 56. I believe it was a

---

[7] *medicinenet.com, 3-21-2018.*

Wednesday. I remember thinking at the time that it might be indigestion from the greasy chili I had for lunch.

The discomfort was enough for me to walk out of class and drive to the emergency room. After some tests, I was admitted to the hospital. Two days later I had a catheter inserted in an artery in my groin, through which the doctor injected dye into the artery going into my heart. He then took images and found significant blockage in the left anterior descending heart artery. He then performed a "rotoblade" procedure. This procedure cleaned the walls of the blocked artery using a catheter inserted in an artery in the groin. They don't do rotoblade any more. He also found 40% blockage of another artery to the heart but did not treat that one.

After the rotoblade procedure, I saw an improvement in my "exercise tolerance." My exercise program at the time was jogging at the high school track. I had kept records of my heart rate relative to running times and pace. I resumed my jogging. It probably was not very smart, but I ran until I felt the pressure in my chest. Then I would slow down enough for it to go away. In about two months my exercise tolerance began to deteriorate.

At my 3 month follow-up with the cardiologist he scheduled me for another catheterization. They found that the same artery was blocked again. The artery was not big enough for a stent. 3 mm was the smallest stent they had at the time. So they just did the "balloon." The balloon expands inside the artery, stretches it, and presses the plaque against the wall of the artery.

The balloon procedure restored my exercise tolerance for two months. Then my exercise tolerance deteriorated again. In October of 1998 Pat drove me to the emergency room with chest pains. I was admitted to the hospital and given a bypass graft of the left mammary artery to the left anterior descending heart artery. Since then I have had no more problems with that artery. I still have the 40% blockage of that other artery.

My heart disease was caused by high cholesterol. My cholesterol and triglycerides were high for a long time before I had any symptoms of heart problems. I believe I could have avoided, or at least delayed, my heart blockage if I had controlled my cholesterol.

It has been almost 20 years since my bypass and my heart blockage doesn't seem to have gotten much worse. I am convinced, it is because my doctor has kept my cholesterol within the recommended guidelines by prescribing statins.

Diet Won't Do It.

After my bypass, I was determined to get my cholesterol in limits. I was sure I could do it with diet and exercise. I was wrong.

All cholesterol comes from animals. There is no cholesterol in plants. I ate nothing but plants for three months between two of my doctor visits. I was trying to avoid going on any more medication. Not only did I not eat animal products, I didn't even eat plant fats such as vegetable oils and margarine. I was a real fat free vegan...a fanatic. It didn't work. My total cholesterol came down a little, but it was still out of limits. My doctor prescribed Crestor®.

After I started taking Crestor® I went back to eating animal products. I tried to keep the red meat down to once or twice a week and eggs just on weekends. But I pretty much ate what I wanted. When I got my next blood test my cholesterol was down. With occasional adjustments to drug type and dosage, my doctor has kept my cholesterol levels close to recommended guidelines for the last 18 years.

Bottom line: My high cholesterol is mostly manufactured by my body and very little comes from what I eat. However, fat bodies tend to produce more cholesterol than lean bodies. Losing weight helped lower my cholesterol.

There are types of cholesterol.

Before we moved to Georgia in 2001, I knew high cholesterol was bad and caused artery blockage. I had heard about LDL and HDL but I didn't know what that meant. After we moved to Georgia, I had to find a new primary healthcare physician. My new doctor started ordering lipid profile analyses that use NMR (Nuclear Magnetic Resonance). This is "...an FDA-cleared blood test...,"[8] that measures cholesterol particle size and concentration. Whereas before we discussed the "good" and "bad" cholesterol levels, now we measured the concentrations of the different particle sizes, the total cholesterol, and triglycerides. LDL (Low Density Lipoproteins) are the large particles and HDL (High Density Lipoproteins) are the small particles. LDLs have been associated with heart disease since the 1950s. Now, with NMR, we can count the LDL particles directly.

The chart on the following page explains it pretty well. You will probably have to go to the web page to read the small print.

---

[8] https://www.labcorp.com/test-menu/32006/nmr-lipoprofile®-without-lipids-with-graph, 3-21-20118.

Understand your NMR lipid profile.[9]

Understanding Your NMR LipoProfile Test Results.

The Science Behind the Test.

Scientists know that heart disease is caused by particles in the blood called low-density lipoproteins, or LDL. But without the tools to measure these LDL particles directly, doctors have traditionally estimated their number by measuring the cholesterol they contain. This measure is known as LDL cholesterol, or LDL-C.

While useful for some patients, knowing the amount of cholesterol in these particles is not as important as knowing the actual number of LDL particles. When high numbers of LDL particles are in the blood, they build up in the arteries and cause heart disease. So a higher number of LDL particles (LDL-P) indicates a higher risk of heart disease.

Highest Risk
High number of small LDL particles

Low Risk
Low number of small LDL particles

- *Cholesterol*
- *LDL Particle*

High number of large LDL particles

Low number of large LDL particles

High Risk

Low Risk

Your LDL-P Number

Your LDL-P number is the most important part of the NMR LipoProfile report. The lower this number is, the less risk you face. In the sample diagram shown below, the relative risk of the LDL-P score is indicated by the highlighted box. The higher your LDL-P number is, the boxes further to the right will be highlighted. As risk goes down, the highlighted box will shift to the left. Your LDL-P number can range from less than 1000 to more than 2000. Based on this number, your doctor can advise you on a treatment plan designed to lower your score to a low-risk level. Your LDL-P goal will depend on your medical history. For example, you may have diabetes or have had a past cardiac event.

LDL-P (LDL Particle Number)	1473 nmol/L	UNDER 1000 Optimal	1000 - 1299 Near or Above Optimal	1300 - 1599 Borderline-High Risk	1600 - 2000 High Risk	OVER 2000 Very High Risk

Your Small LDL-P Number

Your Small LDL-P number is a measure of the number of small LDL particles in your blood. These particles are associated with an increased risk of heart disease; more of these small particles lead to greater risk. Your Small LDL particle score can vary widely, with a lower score being much better. Patients are generally at lower risk for heart disease if their Small LDL-P is less than 700. Patients are at the lowest risk when both their LDL-P number and their Small LDL-P number are low. Your doctor will look at both of these numbers to determine your heart disease risk and to develop a treatment plan for you.

Small LDL-P
950 nmol/L

950
700 SAFE MAXIMUM

Treatment Considerations

Your doctor will help you interpret your NMR LipoProfile test results. If your test results show an increased risk of heart disease, then your doctor may discuss various options with you to lower your risk. These options often include lifestyle changes, such as increased exercise and changes in diet. In some cases your doctor may recommend one or more medications, which may be effective in lowering your LDL-P and Small LDL-P numbers.

Your doctor may choose from these commonly prescribed medications to lower your LDL-P and Small LDL-P numbers:

Class of Drug	Brand Names
Statins	Crestor®, Pravachol®, Lescol XL®, Lipitor®, Zocor®
Niacin	Niaspan®, Niaspan ER®
Fibrates	TriCor®, Lopid®
Cholesterol Absorption Inhibitors	Zetia®

[9] www.nhfcpepicentre.org/Portals/67/docs/
understanding_lipid_profile.pdf, 3-21-2018.

One other thing measured in the LipoProfile is the amount of Triglycerides.

"...an ester formed from glycerol and three fatty acid groups. Triglycerides are the main constituents of natural fats and oils, and high concentrations in the blood indicate an elevated risk of stroke [and heart disease]."[10]

Here is an example of the information from my NMR LipoProfile results of October, 2015.

Report	Result	Ref. Range	Units
LDL-P	866	<1000	NMOL/L
LDL-C	77	0-99	MG/DL
HDL-C	57	>39	MG/DL
TRIGLYCERIDES	93	0-149	MG/DL
TOTAL CHOL.	153	100-199	MG/DL
HDL-P (TOTAL)	35.4	>=30.5	UMOL/L
SMALL LDL-P	398	<=527	NMOL/L
LDL SIZE	20.9	>20.5	NM

---

[10] Google Chrome dictionary, 3-21-2018.

The report also includes interpretative information, including percentile distribution of the particle size and concentrations in "reference population." For example:

Small LDL-P percentile distribution

low	25th	50th	75th	high
<117	117	527	839	>839

4. Diets

My Advice

Do not diet.

Make a short list of food to avoid.

Deviate from your list on rare and special occasions.

Eat 35 grams of fiber every day.

Eat about four times per day in sensible portions.

Diets don't work because the first thing you do on a diet is make a list of stuff to eat. You focus on food.

Diets don't work. Everyone knows you can lose weight by going on a diet. But I challenge you to think of someone who went on a diet and stayed on it the rest of their life. I know people who stayed on a diet for 1 ½ years. I stayed on the Adkins diet for almost a year and lost 30 pounds. But I gained it all back. Usually people will stay on a diet a month or less before going back to their regular lifestyle.

So, what is the answer to controlling your weight?

Quit focusing on food. Everyone I know who went on a diet started off by making a list of things to eat! What you should do is make a short list of foods to avoid.

Here is a "Short List" for you to try:

SUGAR
ANIMAL FAT
FAST FOOD
PROCESSED MEAT
PREPARED MEALS.

Adopt a life style that is healthy and practical. By practical I mean a lifestyle that you can follow every day indefinitely.

Giving up sugar is healthy and practical. It is practical because of its simplicity: "If it has **sugar** don't eat it." Of course "no sugar" means I can never eat dessert. I can never eat ice cream or candy or pie or cake. But it is even bigger than that. There are many sugars: fructose, dextrose, maltose, corn syrup, sucrose, lactose, and more. I cannot drink orange juice. I can eat an orange, but orange juice is a concentration of sugar. Orange juice has 23 grams of sugar per eight ounce serving. I cannot drink milk. Whole milk (4%) has 12 grams of sugar (lactose) per eight ounce serving. I can eat an apple but I cannot drink apple juice. I can eat fresh berries with whipped cream (unsweetened). I know! Whipped cream is loaded cholesterol.

I am not a fan of artificial sweeteners. I use Splenda® on occasion, but I prefer to do without sweets rather than substitute something artificial. Also, there are indications that artificial sweeteners are not healthy.

I have two exceptions to the *no sugar* rule: bread and beer. I love bread and I love beer. I love to make beer, and I love to make bread. I have never had high blood sugar as a result of eating bread or drinking beer.

FYI, I avoid white bread. I prefer whole wheat and grain bread for the fiber, and for the better taste and texture.

Why is it that I can eat bread and drink beer? Because, bread and beer both have yeast in the process. Yeast eats the sugar and gives off alcohol and carbon dioxide. In bread there is about 3 grams of sugar per slice in the making and even though it isn't all eaten by the yeast, the yeast eats enough to get the sugar under my 2 gram per serving guideline. Beer is almost all sugar (maltose) in the making, but the yeast eats it all. There are about 100 calories in the form of complex carbohydrates in a lite beer or in a serving of bread. The healthy body doesn't have any problem handling normal amounts of complex carbs.

I never deviate from the "no sugar" rule. As to the animal fat, fast food, processed food, and prepared meals there may be rare occasions when I might deviate from the rule for social reasons such as special gatherings. It's about your balance of enjoying the moment versus focusing on the future. You have to make some memories.

Enjoy Cooking.
Find the pleasure in creating delicious and healthy meals from natural, unprocessed ingredients. Find the reward in sharing the preparation and eating of a meal with your family.

Leptin resistance may contribute to being overweight.
Leptin Resistance is believed to be the number one cause of people eating too much. Leptin is the hormone that tells the brain when you have enough fat, thus controlling hunger. Leptin **resistance** keeps your brain from getting the message.

"What Science Knows About Reversing Leptin Resistance

The best way to know if you are leptin resistant, is to look in the mirror. If you have a lot of body fat, especially in the belly area, then you are almost certainly leptin resistant.

A key to preventing (or reversing) leptin resistance, is reducing diet-induced inflammation.

There are several things you can do:

Avoid processed food: Highly processed foods may compromise the integrity of the gut and drive inflammation.

Eat Soluble Fiber: Eating soluble fiber can help improve gut health and may protect against obesity.

Exercise: Physical activity may help to reverse leptin resistance.

Sleep: Poor sleep has been implicated in problems with leptin.

Lower your triglycerides: Having high blood triglycerides can prevent the transport of leptin from blood and into the brain. The best way to lower triglycerides is to reduce carbohydrate intake.

Eat Protein: Eating plenty of protein can cause automatic weight loss. There are many reason for that, one of them may be an improvement in leptin sensitivity.

Any of these look familiar? These happen to be many of the same things we generally associate with good health.

Unfortunately, there is no simple way to do this. Eating real food, maintaining a healthy gut, exercising, sleeping well, etc... these are all lifelong endeavours that require a drastic shift in lifestyle." [11]

---

[11] www.healthline.com/nutrition/leptin-101#section7, 3-21-2018.

Fiber is very important.

Eat at least 30 grams of fiber every day. I do this by eating a cup of Fiber One ® cereal every morning, without milk, with blueberries and pecans. This gives me 26 grams of insoluble fiber and a couple of grams of soluble fiber.

Eating insoluble fiber will avoid constipation and the resulting hemorrhoids, diverticulosis, polyps, and increased risk of colon cancer.

Soluble fiber lowers cholesterol, helps control blood sugar levels, and aids in maintaining healthy weight.

I found the following quoted material using Google.

Dietary fiber is material from plant cells that cannot be broken down by enzymes in the human digestive tract. There are two important types of fiber: water-soluble and water insoluble. Each has different properties and characteristics.

- **Soluble** – Water-soluble fibers absorb water during digestion. They increase stool bulk and may decrease blood cholesterol levels. Soluble fiber can be found in fruits (such as apples, oranges and grapefruit), vegetables, legumes (such as dry beans, lentils and peas), barley, oats and oat bran.

- **Insoluble** – Water-insoluble fibers remain unchanged during digestion. They promote normal movement of intestinal contents. Insoluble fiber can be found in fruits with edible peel or seeds, vegetables, whole grain products (such as whole-wheat bread, pasta and crackers), bulgur wheat, stone ground corn meal, cereals, bran, rolled oats, buckwheat and brown rice.[12]

------

[12] https://www.mayoclinic.org/healthy-lifestyle/nutrition-and-healthy-eating/in-depth/fiber/art-20043983, 3-21-2018.

The American Heart Association Eating Plan suggests eating a variety of food fiber sources. Total dietary fiber intake should be 25 to 30 grams a day from food, not supplements. Currently, dietary fiber intakes among adults in the United States average about 15 grams a day. That's about half the recommended amount.

Another benefit attributed to dietary fiber is prevention of colorectal cancer. However, the evidence that fiber reduces colorectal cancer is mixed.[13]

---

[13] https://www.ucsfhealth.org/education/increasing_fiber_intake, 3-21-2018.

5. Exercise

My Advice

Do aerobic exercise at least 30 minutes every day.

Take up a conditioning sport that you enjoy and get good at it.

I have always found a way to get some exercise in my schedule. It has been rewarding. Sometimes it sucked at the time I was doing it, but you have to do something that sucks every day. It makes the rest of the day so much more enjoyable.

These are sports I have enjoyed.

Jogging

I was a runner (jogger is more accurate) for a large part of my adult life. I got my aerobics and some social enjoyment on weekends at 5Ks and 10 Ks. Now I can't run much because of old knees and back pain. But I still walk fast enough to get aerobic benefits.

Hiking

I enjoy walking in the woods. I day hike at Montreat and I have hiked several sections of the AT (Appalachian Trail), backpacking for a week at a time.

Racquetball

I really enjoyed racquetball a lot when I played. It is fast and fun. It takes an hour, you sweat a lot, and it is aerobic. I would still play if it were convenient, but there aren't any courts near where I live.

Tennis

I tried tennis and I liked it ok, but not as much as racquetball. It's great for aerobics and it can be very competitive. If you can afford it, you might enjoy the social aspects of joining a tennis club. Tennis is a sport you can enjoy even after you get old. In your 40s you will switch from singles to doubles. Mixed doubles can put a strain on a marriage, I hope you know.

Weightlifting

I lift weights. I made a talk about weightlifting at a Toastmasters meeting one time. It was about the three different types of weight lifting. They are: bodybuilding, power lifting, and endurance/conditioning. To describe the three types of weightlifting I will need to define "routine," "set," and "rep."

"Routine" is the set of exercises that you do in a weightlifting session. A "Rep" (repetition) is the performance of one exercise one time. A "set" is the performance of several reps of an exercise. For example, curl is an exercise. You might do 24 curls broken up into three sets of 8 reps each.

Now, as to the three types of weightlifting, all three types build strength, muscle mass, and endurance/conditioning. The difference is only in the effort to maximize one of these benefits.

A power lifter who wants to maximize gains in strength will do **high sets** and **low reps.** First she will do a few reps with an easy weight to warm up and stretch. Then she will go to about 80% of what she believes to be her maximum weight and do two reps. Then she will add a plate and do one or two reps. Then she will add a plate and do one or two reps. When she feels she is getting close to her maximum she may just do one rep at each weight. She rests between attempts and works close to the maximum weight she can lift.

Body builders who want to maximize gains in muscle mass and muscle tone will do several sets of eight to twelve reps. Some may prefer to do sets of four to six. But the goal will be to work with weight where you can only lift it a few times. I know one body builder who warms up with 20 to 40 reps of a light weight, then doubles the weight and does four reps. He then adds or removes plates so he stays where he can only do it four times. He doesn't rest more than half a minute between sets so he soon has to start taking off plates so he can still do four. He does about eight sets like this. He calls it "Finding your fours."

Athletes who want to maximize endurance and conditioning will do one (maybe two) sets of high reps with low weight. Some examples are: 40 pushups, 80 sit-ups, 20 benchpresses, or 20 squats.

Biking

I have enjoyed biking since I was ten when I won a brand new Schwinn cruiser with knee action front suspension, tank, horn, headlight, and whitewall tires. I won it at the movie theater one Saturday during the intermission between the two main features.

I beat out a whole stage full of kids performing my skills on the "Toss Top" after only two days of practice. My sister took second place...a pair of roller skates. I had that bike until I was 14 and got a 3-speed English bike. I took long rides on the 3-speed. I rode from White Oak to Possum Creek to go camping. I rode from White Oak across the dam and back home through Chattanooga. I rode a lot until I got a car.

Later I had ten speed road bikes and then 18 speed trail bikes and 21 speed trail bikes. Riding road bikes is good conditioning exercise, and if you like, you can wear those tight pants that show off your junk.

Downhill trail riding is for the young and agile. It really is good for upper body strength due to putting all that weight on your arms. I tried it but it is too hard and dangerous for an old man. Now I just take bikes to the beach when we go camping, or ride on trails made on old railroad beds so there aren't any steep grades. There is a good one near Damascus, Virginia. Also, The Beltway in Atlanta and the trails in Charlotte, are flat and there are no cars.

Golf

I used to walk and carry my clubs. 18 holes of golf is about 5 miles. I walked several times a week when there was a cheap course nearby, but it closed. Now I don't walk when I play golf, because the guy I play with doesn't walk. I primarily get my exercise at the gym.

6. Drive Safely

My Advice

Plan ahead to not drive when you go out to drink.

Observe traffic laws.

Don't tailgate.

Be courteous.

Stay focused.

When you know you are going to be drinking, plan ahead and don't drive. Use Uber® or designate a driver.

Drive the speed limit. I drive about 3 mph over the speed limit on the interstate. But, in Atlanta I drive 70 on the freeway because everyone else does and other drivers get mad if I drive slower.

But, I don't tailgate. I learned when I was a truck driver that following too closely greatly increases your risk of having an accident. It makes you tense and adds stress to your trip, and it can trigger road rage in the person you are following. Not only is it unsafe, it is discourteous.

Be courteous. Let people in. Give them plenty of room. Learn to merge. I have a joke about "the merge gene." Some people can merge and some people can't. Which are you? A safe, courteous driver will never do anything that might cause another driver to have to take an evasive action, i.e. turn, speed up, or slow down.

Oh, and of course, don't text and drive. Put your phone down and focus on driving. Two hands on the wheel.

Check your mirrors every few seconds. Know who is in your blind spot at all times.

Be aware of whether you have an escape route in case some other driver does something unexpected. If there is no shoulder, slow down and open more room between you and the cars ahead.

> "Accidents, also referred to as unintentional injuries, are at present the 4th leading cause of death in the US and the leading cause of death for those aged1-44.[14]"

In 2016 in the US, over 37,000 deaths resulted from automobile accidents. Automobile accidents are the number one cause of death for young people.

---

[14] Hannah Nichols, https://www.medicalnewstoday.com/articles/282929.php, 3-21-2018.

7. Your Family History

My Advice

Know your family health history.

Take preventive/corrective action for high risk issues.

Here is a list of the health issues on my side of your family:

- Pernicious anemia
- Coronary artery blockage (high cholesterol)
- Cancer
- Type II diabetes
- Hypothyroidism
- Polyps of the colon
- Anxiety
- High Blood Pressure
- Leukemia
- Lymphoma
- Parkinson's disease

Pernicious anemia is caused by vitamin B-12 deficiency. In the 1940s, it was untreatable and resulted in a slow death from nerve deterioration. Now it is treated with a B-12 injection once per month. It is not curable, but it is easily treated. I have pernicious anemia and I give myself a shot on the first of every month.

My father also had pernicious anemia, but since I didn't have contact with my father, I didn't know about it. As a result, I was not diagnosed until I was almost completely paralyzed below the waist.

My first symptoms appeared when I was about 49 years old. The early symptoms include being tired and numbness in the fingers and toes. Later, there was loss of use of my legs. Also, when I moved my head to look down, touching my chin to my chest, I would experience a tingling, like an electric shock, down my back. This was caused by the inflammation of my spinal column.

If you have any of these symptoms, let your doctor know this runs in your family. My doctor used the **Schillings Test** to confirm that I had pernicious anemia.

Coronary artery blockage and type II diabetes are discussed in previous chapters.

My skin cancer was a squamous cell carcinoma on my left hand. It was probably the result of sun damage.

Hypothyroidism started when I was in my late 60s. I take a pill every day. My dosage kept increasing over several years. In the Fall of 2017 my dosage was reduced a little. Kelley (my daughter) says you need less as you get older.

I have had polyps of the colon removed on two occasions during routine colonoscopies. Eat your fiber. Don't take aspirin for two weeks after you have a polyp removed. I had to have four units of blood because I took aspirin.

Anxiety is a feeling of dread. It is a feeling that something really bad is about to happen. I have had it for most of my adult life. I don't want to speculate about what causes it. I just want to say what works for me in dealing with anxiety.

I took Lexapro® for a few years. It helped a lot. I seemed to feel less stress. I exhibited less anger. The side effects didn't seem very obvious. I may have had less motivation to do things, and there may have been some loss of sexual interest. If so, these effects were very minor.

I stopped taking Lexapro® by replacing it with hard aerobic exercise. At the same time that I was reducing my dosage, I started doing a full hour of aerobic exercise every day. I would walk on a treadmill or use the recumbent bicycle. I got my heart rate to about 80% of maximum and kept it there for the remainder of the hour. I can tell you for sure, in my case, an hour of hard exercise is as good as a pill for helping with anxiety.

I first experienced high blood pressure when I was in my 70s. My doctor prescribed Losartan.

> Losartan... is used to treat high blood pressure (hypertension). It's also used to lower the risk of stroke in some patients with heart disease. Losartan is an angiotensin receptor blocker (ARB) that blocks a substance that causes blood vessels to tighten. By relaxing blood vessels, losartan helps a person maintain a lower blood pressure, increasing the supply of oxygen and blood to the heart. Losartan is also used to slow long-term kidney damage for people with type 2 diabetes, and it is sometimes used to treat congestive heart failure.[15]

---

[15] https://www.everydayhealth.com/drugs/losartan, 4-22-2018.

Generally the people in my family have lived into their late seventies or early eighties.

My Parents:

- Marvin Russell Walker was born November 1919. He died around 2011 at the age of 92. He had coronary blockage and pernicious anemia.
- Annie Ella Hill Walker was born January 10, 1918. She died December 23, 1963, at the age of 45. She suffered a blood clot following hysterectomy surgery.

My Father's Parents:

- George Washington Walker was born in 1897. He died in his early 80s, I don't know the cause of death.
  The 1910 census records him and his sister Molly living in Graysville, Tennessee, with a family whose last name was Rudd. So he was 13 at the time. George's father, James Walker, lived in the same community, actually on the same road. George's Mother was half Cherokee. I don't know her name or how she died. After she died, James married Amy (Maiden name Dowker). Amy had a daughter, Lizzie Marie, from a previous marriage. George went out on his own at the age of 16. The people in the community called him "Walker's Injun." George later married Lizzie Marie, his step sister.

- Lizzie Marie died giving birth to a daughter, their seventh child. The baby also died.
  George then married Martha. All the Walker boys frowned at the mention of her name. They all left home at an early age. Mart (Martha) had three boys, Curtis, Jack, and Casto Smith. The Smith boys still lived at home long after they were grown. My dad said about Mart and her two sisters: "They's any man's dog that'd hunt 'em."

My Mother's Parents:

- John Meyer Hill was born September 19, 1896. He died in 1974 at the age of 78. He was cutting grass for his son Charles. He came inside and said: "I need to lie down." He had a heart attack and died.
- Mattie Dowker Hill was born December 7, 1889. She died in 1960 at the age of 71 due to a blood clot to her heart following minor surgery.

My parents were cousins (Soddy ain't no big place):

There were three Dowker sisters: Amy, Bertha and Mattie. Amy was Lizzie Marie's mother and Russell's Grandmother. Mattie was Annie's mother. They tell me that makes my parents "First cousins once removed."

Bertha had one adopted daughter, Lucille. Lucille raised Mandy, my half sister, except for about three years when Mandy was 10 to 12 years old and she lived with us.

My siblings:

- My Sister Mandy (Madeline Hill Akers) was born June 9, 1939. We have different fathers. At one time she thought she had found out who her father was. But her DNA ancestry results have cast doubt in her mind due to the absence of Native American markers for her. She is still living. She has a history of heart blockage which she manages with diet. She underwent chemo therapy for lymphoma in 2007. She remained cancer free for nine years. In February of 2018 her lymphoma returned and she is now undergoing another round of chemotherapy.
- My Brother, Pepper (Guinn Lafayette Walker) was born December 2, 1942. He died of a heart attack in his mid sixties.
- My Brother Marvin Russell Walker III was born December 12, 1948. He died of diabetes and kidney failure in his mid sixties.

Here is a diagram that might help with the aforementioned relations:

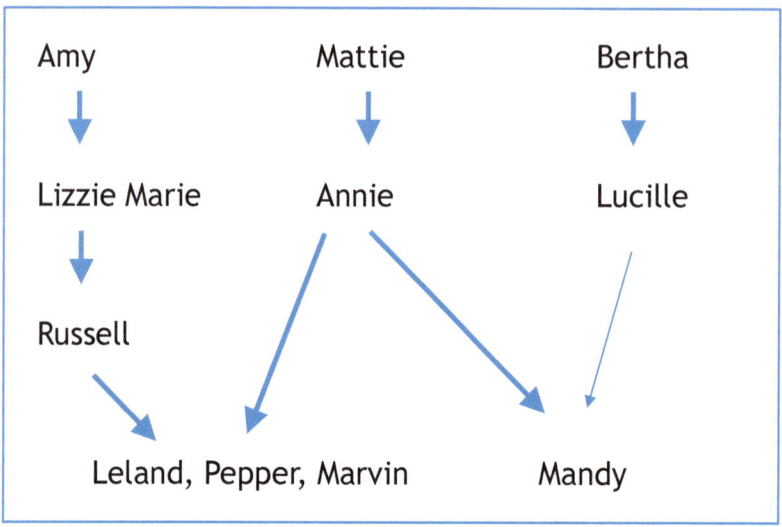

My Father had five brothers and one sister.

- James Lee was born 9/23/2017 and died 1/21/1994. He had diabetes and then kidney failure and was on dialysis. He also had arthritis. He smoked in his earlier years but quit. He had some issues while he was on dialysis with fluid gathering in his chest that had to be drained.
- Homer had a stroke in his 80s and died a year or two later. Homer had a happy nature. He loved to sing old obscure country songs. He sang loudly and played guitar poorly. Even when he was paralyzed by the stroke he could still display a big happy smile. Homer didn't believe in whipping his kids. He said it just makes them grow up fearing and hating. His wife Pet, on the other hand, just about killed an apple tree cutting switches off of it.
- Aunt Neoma, Mattie Naomi Walker Atchley, died of heart failure in her 80s. She also had Parkinson's disease. I stayed with her for a week

in the summer on two occasions when I was about 12. Her son Charles was two years younger than me but he could whip me. Aunt Neoma could throw a rock like a man. Once she threw a rock at one of her husband's guineas to get it out of her garden and accidentally killed it. She never told him. Just before she died she was in the hospital attached to a defibrillator. She got tired of it shocking her and told them: "If that is the best y'all can do you can just send me home." They did. I saw her at her son's house before she died. Uncle Wendell and Uncle Howard were there. We all laughed about my dad being a Jehovah's Witness.

- Uncle Eugene was in the Navy. He came home from WWII with "Shell Shock." He was always nervous and his speech was not real smooth. But he wasn't shy. He was personable and friendly. He had a nerve problem. It may have been Parkinson's.
- Uncle Howard died at 76. He had lung cancer and had just completed chemotherapy and had started radiation treatments to the brain. He started having mini strokes and slipped into a coma and passed. He had no diabetes. He was always thin. He was anemic, perhaps he had pernicious anemia. Uncle Howard was a gentle man and didn't talk much. My dad took Howard's wife Jean and two sons away from him and beat him up. He then raised Howard's boys to be Jehovah's Witnesses. Howard remarried and had two fine boys and a step-daughter. Jean didn't stay with my dad. She left him for someone else. You know what Dr. Phil says: "If they'll do it **with** you, they'll do it **to** you."
- Uncle Wendell died at 82 from lymphoma. He was my favorite. People said we looked alike. I remember when he went to war at the age of 18. He fought in trenches in Korea. He returned home, bought a brand new 1954 Ford Crowned Victoria, and married the prettiest girl in the Soddy Ridges...Thelma Penny.

My Mother had two brothers and two sisters:

- Charles Wallace Hill was born May 22, 1925. He died of leukemia in November 1999. It was a slow progressing type of leukemia. He had it for several years before he died. Charles and Judy adopted two children: Joanie and Dickie. Uncle Charles was a hard working and friendly guy. He was confident and self assured. My favorite memory is the Sunday dinner yeast rolls rising on top of their refrigerator.
- Lillie Bernice Hill Gray was born August 8, 1919. She died around 2013. Tippy said she died of old age. When I last saw her on one of my sailing trips she was having memory problems. Later I heard she had dementia. Aunt Lillie was a gracious host when I visited. She married a Navy pilot and had four children who are all very smart, good looking, and successful. She and her Navy Captain are buried at Arlington National Cemetery. I am fortunate to have attended both ceremonies
- Glendean Louise Hill Bottom was born July 26, 1927. She died in 2006 of cancer. I got to spend a week at her basement apartment when I was 10. Her husband Ernie was selling shoes and going to night school to finish his degree. Ernie was grumpy but Dean was wonderful. She played games with Mandy and me, and made my favorite pie...pecan! Dean (Glendean) talked Ernie into taking me to town for my first ride on an escalator. When Dean died, I flew to Seattle. On the return flight Mandy and I were on the same plane from Seattle to Denver. That is the only time I know of Mandy being on a plane.
- John Meyer Hill (Tippy) was born June 19, 1931. He assures me he has not died yet. He had a triple coronary bypass in 2003. He has type II diabetes with complications causing him to have "mini-strokes" and poor circulation. He is about to have surgery to improve the circulation to his legs. He has diabetic neuropathy (high blood sugar - glucose - can injure nerve fibers throughout your body, but diabetic

neuropathy most often damages nerves in your legs and feet)[16]. Diabetic neuropathy can cause pain or numbness. Tip is having pain.

---

[16] https://www.mayoclinic.org/diseases-conditions/ diabetic-neuropathy/symptoms-causes/syc-20371580, 4-22-2018.

8. Professional Healthcare

I have excellent healthcare. My primary care physician has managed to keep my cholesterol controlled so that I have not had a recurrence of heart blockage. I take five drugs that keep me alive and healthy and one drug that keeps me happy.

My Advice

Select a primary healthcare physician that you trust.

Take an active role in your healthcare decisions.

Be knowledgable. Just Google it.

Be proactive. Practice preventive medicine.

Get professional help when you need it.

ABOUT THE AUTHOR

Leland Walker lives in Jonesboro, Georgia with his wife Pat, their dog Frank, and their cat Tuxedo. Leland has eleven grandchildren, and two great-nephews who are the same as grandchildren.

www.ingramcontent.com/pod-product-compliance
Lightning Source LLC
Chambersburg PA
CBHW050824290526
45792CB00001B/245